YOUR KNOWLEDGE HAS VALUE

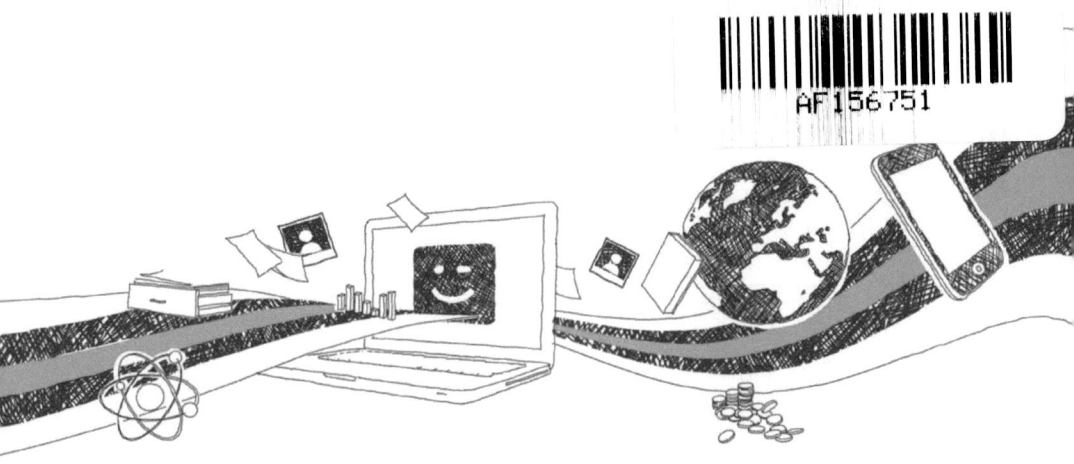

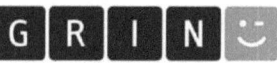

Bibliographic information published by the German National Library:

The German National Library lists this publication in the National Bibliography; detailed bibliographic data are available on the Internet at http://dnb.dnb.de .

Imprint:

Copyright © 2012 GRIN Verlag
Print and binding: Books on Demand GmbH, Norderstedt Germany
ISBN: 9783346104151

Ojo Rotimi

Alcoholism. Causes, Effects and Treatments

GRIN Verlag

GRIN - Your knowledge has value

Since its foundation in 1998, GRIN has specialized in publishing academic texts by students, college teachers and other academics as e-book and printed book. The website www.grin.com is an ideal platform for presenting term papers, final papers, scientific essays, dissertations and specialist books.

Visit us on the internet:

http://www.grin.com/

http://www.facebook.com/grincom

http://www.twitter.com/grin_com

Table of Contents

INTRODUCTION

History

Historically the name dipsomania was coined by German physician C. W. Hufeland in 1819 before it was superseded by alcoholism. [1] The term "alcoholism" was first used in 1849 by the Swedish physician Magnus Huss to describe the systematic adverse effects of alcohol. [2]

Alcohol has a long history of use and misuse throughout recorded history. Biblical, Egyptian and Babylonian sources record the history of abuse and dependence on alcohol. In some ancient cultures alcohol was worshiped and in others its abuse was condemned. Excessive alcohol misuse and drunkenness were recognised as causing social problems.

The various health problems associated with long-term alcohol consumption are generally perceived as detrimental to society, for example, money due to lost labor-hours, medical costs, and secondary treatment costs. Alcohol use is a major contributing factor for head injuries, motor vehicle accidents, violence, and assaults. Beyond money, there are also significant social costs to both the alcoholic and their family and friends. [3] For instance, alcohol consumption by a pregnant woman can lead to fetal alcohol syndrome. Alcoholism is a primary chronic disease characterized by addiction to alcohol.

Definition

Alcoholism is a broad term for problems with alcohol, and is generally used to mean compulsive and uncontrolled consumption of alcoholic beverages, usually to the detriment of the drinker's health, personal relationships, and social standing. It is medically considered a disease, specifically a neurological disorder, and in medicine several other terms are used, specifically "alcohol abuse" and "alcohol dependence," which have more specific definitions. Peoples suffering from alcoholism are often called "alcoholic". The World Health Organization estimates that there are 140 million people with alcoholism worldwide. [4]

Alcoholism is called a "dual disease" since it includes both mental and physical components. The biological mechanisms that cause alcoholism are not well understood. Social environment, stress, mental health, family history, age, ethnic group, and gender all influence the risk for the condition. Alcohol damages almost every organ in the body, including the brain. The cumulative toxic effects of chronic alcohol abuse can cause both medical and psychiatric problems. [5] Identifying alcoholism is difficult for the individual afflicted because of the social stigma associated with the disease that causes people with alcoholism to avoid diagnosis and treatment for fear of shame or social consequences.

Alcohol

What is alcohol? *Alcohol* is a general term for any organic compound in which a hydroxyl group (-O H) is bound to a carbon atom, which in turn may be bound to other carbon atoms and further hydrogens. Alcohols other than ethanol (such as propylene glycol and the sugar alcohols) appear in food and beverages.

The concept of this seminar is based on alcohol beverage. Alcohol (also known as ethyl alcohol or ethanol) is the principal product of fermentation. In this process, yeast cells act on the sugar content of fruits and grains to produce alcohol and carbondioxide.

An **alcoholic beverage** is a drink containing ethanol, commonly known as alcohol. Alcoholic beverages are divided into three general classes: beers, wines, and spirits. They are legally consumed in most countries, and over 100 countries have laws regulating their production, sale, and consumption. In particular, such laws specify the minimum age at which a person may legally buy or drink them.

This minimum age varies between 16 and 25 years, depending upon the country and the type of drink. Most nations set it at 18 years of age.

The production and consumption of alcohol occurs in most cultures of the world, from hunter-gatherer peoples to nation-states. Alcoholic beverages are often an important part of social events in these cultures.

Alcohol is a psychoactive drug that has a depressant effect. A high blood alcohol content is usually considered to be legal drunkenness because it reduces attention and slows reaction speed. In some countries such as Sweden public drinking of alcohol are banned and while some Muslim countries, such as Saudi Arabia , Kuwait, Sudan , Pakistan, Iran, and Libya prohibit production, sale and consumption of alcohol beverages because they are forbidden by Islam. In Denmark, Netherlands, it is generally legal to drink alcoholic beverages in the street.

Types of alcohol beverage

1. Wine

2. Beer

3. Distillation/ spirit

WINE: - Wine is made from the fermented juice of grapes or other fruits, it has a typical alcohol content of 10% to 14% by volume. There are five basic types of wine, which are Red, White, Rose and sparkling or champ ague, containing carbondioxide (all referred to as table wine)and dessert for cocktail (with an alcohol content ranging from 15% to 24%).

BEER:-They are derived from cereal grains a barley, rye, corn and wheat. The process of making is referred to as brewing and include the conversion of cereal and starch to fermentable sugar and it is then stored. The typical alcohol content is about 4%. Light beers are about 3.2% to 3.3% alcohol.

DISTILLED BEVERAGES:-This are wines and beers subjected to other process to increase their alcoholic content by heating them collected into a reservoir when it turns back into liquid form, the ends product is distilled spirits. Alcohol content of distilled beverage is about 40% and 50% volume.

Local alcohol beverage in Nigeria

1. Local Gin: ogogoro, kia kia, Akparin (got by distilled palm wine)

2. Oguro: (got from Rafia palm)

3. Palm wine: (got from the oil palm tree)

Uses of alcohol

Alcohol is used for different purposes which include; social, medical, dietary, mood modification, entertainment, laboratory work, and peacemaking.

Why people use or abuse alcohol

Alcoholic beverages have been drunk by people around the world since ancient times. Reasons that have been proposed for drinking them include:

1. To cope with family problems

2. To be able to work better

3. To change their mood

4. To get high

6

5. To ease pain

6. To be cool

7. To hurt themselves

8. They are part of a people's standard diet

9. They are drunk for medical reasons

10. For their relaxant effects

11. For their euphoric effects

12. For recreational purposes

13. For artistic inspiration

14. For their putative aphrodisiac effects

Factors that influence alcohol abuse

A complex mixture of genetic and environmental factors influences the risk of the development of alcoholism.

Genetic factor

Genes that influence the metabolism of alcohol also influence the risk of alcoholism, and may be indicated by a family history of alcoholism. One paper has found that alcohol use at an early age may influence the expression of genes which increase the risk of alcohol dependence. Individuals who have a genetic disposition to alcoholism are also more likely to begin drinking at an earlier age than average.[6]

Environmental factor

Home and family; alcohol abuse begin in childhood is often associated with the home and family. Children seem to be at greater risk when parents exhibit poor management skill, anti social behavior. Others are school, peers group and community.

Modeling and advertisements; children and adolescences are frequently exposé to beer and liquor advertising. In the process of advertising, children, adolescent and adult usually think that alcohol consumption is good to health.

Symptoms of alcoholism

1. Anxiety and depression
2. Craving (a strong need or to drink alcohol)
3. Lost of control (not being able to stop drinking once drinking begins)
4. Physical dependence (withdrawal symptom such as nausea, sweating, shakiness and anxiety after stop drinking)

5. To tolerance (the need for drinking greater amount of alcohol for the same effect)

EFFECTS OF ALCOHOL

The possible effects of alcohol maybe physical, psychiatric and social.

Alcoholism is characterized by an increased tolerance of and physical dependence on alcohol, affecting an individual's ability to control alcohol consumption safely. These characteristics are believed to play a role in impeding an alcoholic's ability to stop drinking. Alcoholism can have adverse effects on mental health, causing psychiatric disorders and increasing the risk of suicide.

Physical effects

Long-term alcohol abuse can cause a number of physical symptoms, including cirrhosis of the liver, pancreatitis, epilepsy, polyneuropathy, alcoholic dementia, heart disease, nutritional deficiencies, peptic ulcers and sexual dysfunction, and can eventually be fatal. Other physical effects include an increased risk of developing cardiovascular disease, malabsorption, alcoholic liver disease, and cancer. Damage to the central nervous system and peripheral nervous system can occur from sustained alcohol consumption. [7]

Women develop long-term complications of alcohol dependence more rapidly than do men. Additionally, women have a higher mortality rate from alcoholism than men. Examples of long-term complications include brain, heart, and liver damage and an increased risk of breast cancer. Additionally, heavy drinking over time has been found to have a negative effect on reproductive functioning in women. This result in reproductive dysfunction such as anovulation, decreased ovarian mass, problems or irregularity of the menstrual cycle, and early menopause. Alcoholic ketoacidosis can occur in individuals who chronically abuse alcohol and have a recent history of binge drinking [13]. Additionally, in pregnant women, alcohol can cause fetal alcohol syndrome.

Psychiatric effects

Long-term misuse of alcohol can cause a wide range of mental health problems. Severe cognitive problems are common; approximately 10 percent of all dementia cases are related to alcohol consumption, making it the second leading cause of dementia. Excessive alcohol use causes damage to brain function, and psychological health can be increasingly affected over time. [8]

Psychiatric disorders are common in alcoholics, with as many as 25 percent suffering severe psychiatric disturbances. The most prevalent psychiatric symptoms are anxiety and depression disorders. Psychosis, confusion, and organic brain syndrome may be caused by alcohol misuse, which can lead to a misdiagnosis such as schizophrenia. Panic disorder can develop or worsen as a direct result of long-term alcohol misuse. Additional use of other drugs may increase the risk of depression. [9]

Psychiatric disorders differ depending on gender. Women who have alcohol-use disorders often have a co-occurring psychiatric diagnosis such as major depression, anxiety, panic disorder, bulimia, post-traumatic stress disorder (PTSD), or borderline personality disorder. Men with alcohol-use disorders more often have a co-occurring diagnosis of narcissistic or antisocial personality disorder, bipolar disorder, schizophrenia, impulse disorders or attention deficit/hyperactivity disorder. Women with alcoholism are more likely to have a history of physical or sexual assault, abuse and domestic violence than those in the general population which can lead to higher instances of psychiatric disorders and greater dependence on alcohol. [10]

Social effects

The social problems arising from alcoholism are serious, caused by the pathological changes in the brain and the intoxicating effects of alcohol. Alcohol abuse is associated with an increased risk of committing criminal offences, including child abuse, domestic violence, rape, burglary and assault. Alcoholism is associated with loss of employment which can lead to financial problems. Drinking at inappropriate times and behavior caused by reduced judgment, can lead to legal consequences, such as criminal charges for drunk driving or public disorder, or civil penalties for tortious behavior, and may lead to a criminal sentence.

An alcoholic's behavior and mental impairment, while drunk, can profoundly affect those surrounding them and lead to isolation from family and friends. This isolation can lead to marital conflict and divorce, or contribute to domestic violence. Alcoholism can also lead to child neglect, with subsequent lasting damage to the emotional development of the alcoholic's children. For this reason, children of alcoholic parents can develop a number of emotional problems. For example, they can become afraid of their parents, because of their unstable mood behaviors. In addition, they can develop considerable amount of shame over their inadequacy to liberate their parents from alcoholism. As a result of this failure, they develop wretched self-images, which can lead to depression.

CONTROL MEASURES

Prevention

The World Health Organization, the European Union and other regional bodies, national governments and parliaments have formed alcohol policies in order to reduce the harm of alcoholism. Targeting adolescents and young adults is regarded as an important step to reduce the harm of alcohol abuse. Increasing the age at which licit drugs of abuse such as alcohol can be purchased, the banning or restricting advertising of alcohol has been recommended as additional ways of reducing the harm of alcohol dependence and abuse. Guidelines for parents to prevent alcohol abuse amongst adolescents and for helping young people with mental health problems have also been suggested. [11]

Treatment

Detoxification

Alcohol detoxification or 'detox' for alcoholics is an abrupt stop of alcohol drinking coupled with the substitution of drugs, such as benzodiazepines, that have similar effects to prevent alcohol withdrawal. Detoxification does not actually treat alcoholism, and it is necessary to follow-up detoxification with an appropriate treatment program for alcohol dependence or abuse in order to reduce the risk of relapse.

Psychological

Various forms of group therapy or psychotherapy can be used to deal with underlying psychological issues that are related to alcohol addiction, as well as provide relapse prevention skills. The mutual-help group-counseling approach is one of the most common ways of helping alcoholics maintain sobriety. Alcoholics Anonymous was one of the first organizations formed to provide mutual, nonprofessional counseling, and it is still the largest. Others include LifeRing Secular Recovery, SMART Recovery, Women For Sobriety, and Secular Organization ns for Sobriety.

Rationing and moderation programs such as Moderation Management and Drink Wise do not mandate complete abstinence. While most alcoholics are unable to limit their drinking in this way, some return to moderate drinking.

Medications

A variety of medications may be prescribed as part of treatment for alcoholism.

- Vitamin supplements (most importantly thiamine)

- Disulfiram (Antabuse) prevents the elimination of acetaldehyde, a chemical the body produces when breaking down ethanol.

- Calcium carbimide (Temposil) works in the same way as disulfiram; it has an advantage in that the occasional adverse effects of disulfiram, hepatotoxicity and drowsiness, do not occur with calcium carbimide. [12]

- Naltrexone is a competitive antagonist for opioid receptors, effectively blocking the effects of endorphins and opiates. Naltrexone is used to decrease cravings for alcohol and encourage abstinence. Alcohol causes the body to release endorphins, which in turn release dopamine and activate the reward pathways; hence when naltrexone is in the body there is a reduction in the pleasurable effects from consuming alcohol.

- Odansetron, a 5HT3 antagonist, is effective in the treatment of alcoholism; the combination of odansetron and naltrexone is superior than either treatment alone.

- Acamprosate (Campral) stabilises the brain chemistry that is altered due to alcohol dependence via antagonising the actions of glutamate, a neurotransmitter which is hyperactive in the post-withdrawal phase. By reducing excessive NMDA activity which occurs at the onset of alcohol withdrawal, acamprosate can reduce or prevent alcohol withdrawal related neurotoxicity

- Benzodiazepines, while useful in the management of acute alcohol withdrawal, if used long-term can cause a worse outcome in alcoholism. Alcoholics on chronic benzodiazepines have a lower rate of achieving abstinence from alcohol than those not taking benzodiazepines. This class of drugs is commonly prescribed to alcoholics for insomnia or anxiety management.

Management

Treatments are varied because there are multiple perspectives of alcoholism. Those who approach alcoholism as a medical condition or disease recommend differing treatments than, for instance, those who approach the condition as one of social choice. Most treatments focus on helping people discontinue their alcohol intake, followed up with life training and/or social support in order to help them resist a return to alcohol use. Since alcoholism involves multiple factors which encourage a person to continue drinking, they must all be addressed in order to successfully prevent a relapse. [14] An example of this kind of treatment is detoxification followed by a combination of supportive therapy, attendance at self-help groups, and ongoing development of coping mechanisms.

CONCLUSION

In conclusion, alcoholism is a chronic diseases caused by alcohol drinks, e.g. cirrhosis, gastritis, pancreatic failure, liver dysfunction, hypertension, fetal alcoholic syndrome, hepatitis, epilepsy, polyneuropathy, alcoholic dementia, heart disease, and cancer (l.e cancer of the mouth, cancer of the tongue, cancer of the esophagus, cancer of the liver, e.t.c), Psychosis, confusion, and organic brain syndrome may be caused by alcohol misuse. Increased risk of developing cardiovascular disease, malabsorption, damage to the central nervous system and peripheral nervous system can occur from sustained alcohol consumption.

Therefore, taken a certain drug that can lead to more than twenty (20) varieties of diseases, this shows the deleterious consequences of alcohol. Thus, in addition, "Health is Wealth". In order to achieve this, it is advisable to avoid excessive alcohol consumption. Prevention is better than cure.

RECOMMENDATIONS

Alcoholism is called a "dual disease" since it includes both mental and physical components. It is recommended that every individual should know how to control alcohol consumptions; you can control alcohol consumption by doing the following;

1. Avoid parties where you can logically expect heavy drinking.
2. Avoid people who used to drinking alcohol heavily.
3. Move with friends who does not drink alcohol
4. Request a non-alcoholic beer, soft drink or glass of water instead of alcohol.

Government should be able to

1. Write to alcohol producers, such as sea grams to voice their concern.
2. Boycott the products of companies that produces alcoholic drinks

3. Write to television and cable stations not advertise or reduces advert that encourage alcohol consumption

4. Boycott programming that supported by alcohol advertising that targets youth.

5. Organize seminars on the effects of alcohol

REFERENCES

1. Peters, Uwe Henrik (30 April 2007). Lexikon Psychiatrie, Psychotherapie, Medizinische Psychologie. Urban Fischer bei Elsev.

2. Alcoholismus chronicus, eller Chronisk alkoholssjukdom:. Stockholm und Leipzig. 1852. http://books.google.com/?id=wt6r2Zw8sCEC&pg=PR5. Retrieved 19 February 2008.

3. McCully, Chris (2004). *Goodbye Mr. Wonderful. Alcohol, Addition and Early Recovery.*. London: Jessica Kingsley Publishers. ISBN 978-1-84310-265-6. http://www.jkp.com/catalogue/book/9781843102656/contents.

4. "Alcohol policy in the WHO European Region: current status and the way forward" (PDF). World Health Organisation. 12 September 2005.

5. Caan, Woody; Belleroche, Jackie de, eds. (11 April 2002). *Drink, Drugs and Dependence: From Science to Clinical Practice* (1st ed.). Routledge. pp. 19–20. ISBN 978-0-415-27891-1.

6. Agarwal-Kozlowski, K.; Agarwal, DP. (Apr 2000). "[Genetic predisposition for alcoholism]". *Ther Umsch* 57 (4): 179–84. PMID 10804873.

7. Testino G (2008). "Alcoholic diseases in hepato-gastroenterology: a point of view". *Hepatogastroenterology* 55 (82–83): 371–7.

8. Oscar-Berman, Marlene; Marinkovic, Ksenija (2003). "Alcoholism and the brain: an overview". *Alcohol Res Health* 27 (2): 125–33. PMID 15303622.

9. Schuckit MA (November 1983). "Alcoholism and other psychiatric disorders". *Hosp Community Psychiatry* **34** (11): 1022–7. ISSN 0022-1597. PMID 6642446.

10. Karrol Brad R. (2002). "Women and alcohol use disorders: a review of important knowledge and its implications for social work practitioners". *Journal of social work* **2** (3): 337–356. DOI:10.1177/146801730200200305.

11. Crews, F.; He, J.; Hodge, C. (Feb 2007). "Adolescent cortical development: a critical period of vulnerability for addiction". *Pharmacol Biochem Behav* **86** (2): 189–99. DOI:10.1016/j.pbb.2006.12.001. PMID 17222895.

12. Ogborne, AC. (June 2000). "Identifying and treating patients with alcohol-related problems". *CMAJ* **162** (12): 1705–8. PMC 1232509. PMID 10870503.

13. Sibaï, K.; Eggimann, P. (Sep 2005). "[Alcoholic ketoacidosis: not rare cause of metabolic acidosis]". *Rev Med Suisse* **1** (32): 2106, 2108–10, 2112–5. PMID 16238232.

14. Wetterling T; Junghanns, K (September 2000). "Psychopathology of alcoholics during withdrawal and early abstinence". *Eur Psychiatry* **15** (8): 483–8. DOI:10.1016/S0924-9338(00)00519-8. ISSN 0924-9338.

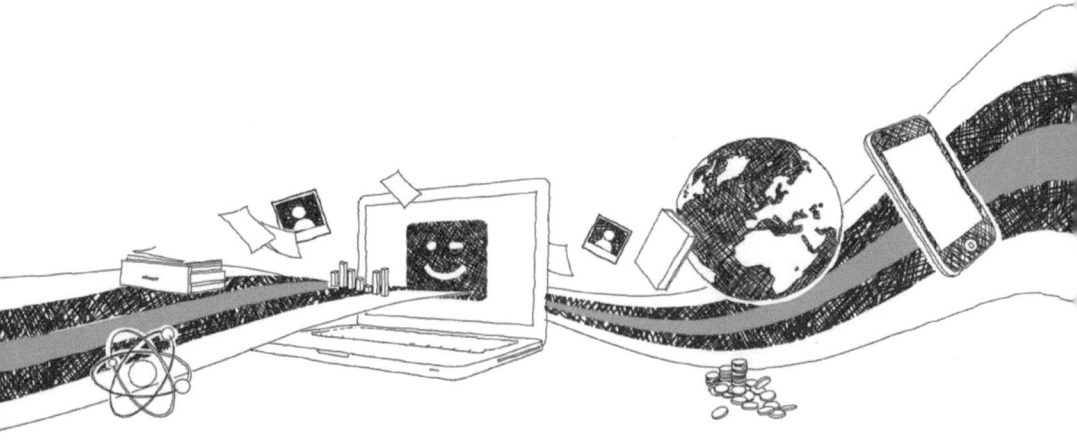
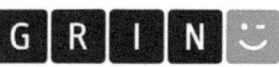